Heart Attack

Written by MARTIN SHARP
Illustrated by JAMES E. BARRY
Designed by MARGO ELL

Delair Consolidated new york
A DELAIR PUBLISHING COMPANY

Delair Publishing Company, Inc.
420 Lexington Avenue,
New York, New York 10017

ISBN: 0-8326-2408-X

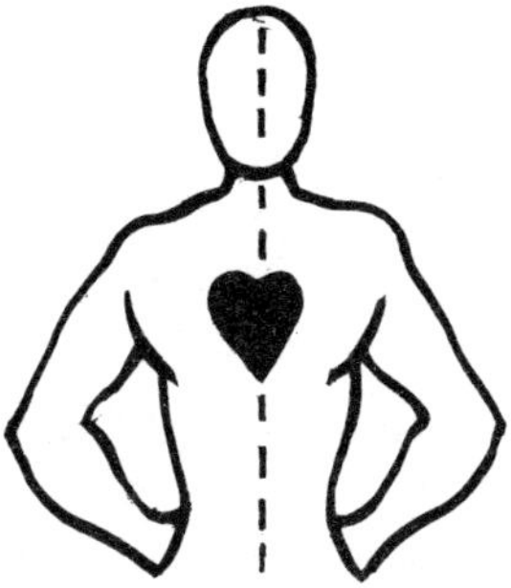

The heart is positioned in the center of the chest.

Heart Attack!

Those two words are frightening to everyone. They mean pain, suffering, fear, financial troubles, and possibly death.

Would you know a heart attack if you had one? Could you tell a heart attack from severe indigestion? Just what is a heart attack, and how does it occur? How can you live a reasonably normal life after a heart attack? These are questions this booklet will answer.

How to Recognize a Heart Attack

Heart attack can strike anyone at any age and at any time. It is important to know the symptoms that signal a heart attack because if it does occur, there is no time for delay in getting medical care.

The pain a heart attack causes is not the same for everybody. One person may feel pain more severely than another. The milder pain is often believed by the victim to be "indigestion." Although the symptoms vary, the usual warnings of a heart attack are the following:

The first symptom is an uncomfortable, heavy, squeezing pain in the center of the chest (that's where your heart is, not on the left as many believe) lasting for several minutes. Sharp, stabbing pains usually do not mean a heart attack.

As the pain becomes worse, it radiates to the left shoulder and down the left arm.

The pain may spread to the right shoulder and arm and to the neck and lower jaw. A sensation of fullness or squeezing may occur in the abdomen. This is often mistaken for indigestion.

Pain may occur in any one or a combination of these areas at the same time. It may even go away and then recur.

In addition to the pain during a heart attack, there may be:

anxiety
sweating
nausea and vomiting
shortness of breath and gasping for air
dizziness and fainting

What do Do If a Heart Attack Does Occur

At the first warning sign act immediately to get help. Don't wait to make sure the symptoms really mean a heart attack. Call a doctor or emergency service without delay. In many communities the emergency telephone number is 911. If you have trouble getting help by phone, go to a hospital or clinic emergency room at once. If you are alone, call a taxi or ask anyone available to take you there. Don't be embarrassed to ask a stranger.

Mouth-to-mouth breathing.

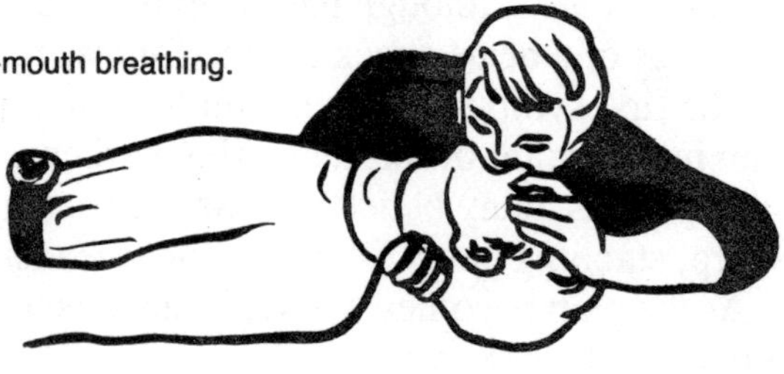

You can give life-saving support to a person whose heart has stopped beating during a heart attack until professional help arrives. You can do this by *cardiopulmonary resuscitation (CPR),* which is mouth-to-mouth breathing plus rhythmic pressure on the chest. Everybody can do mouth-to-mouth breathing, but compressing the chest should be done only by specially trained persons. Training in CPR is available through local chapters of the American Heart Association and the American Red Cross.

The Heart

To understand heart attacks, it is necessary to understand how the heart works.

The heart is a muscle about the size of a fist. It is hollow and is divided into two chambers on each side. A thin, solid wall of tissue separates the left side from the right. The upper chambers are called *atria* (or *auricles*); the lower are *ventricles.* Valves connect the atria and the ventricles. The valves operate only one way—from the upper heart chambers to the lower. Blood enters the heart through a large vein called the *vena cava,* which opens into the right atrium. The blood has come to the vena cava from all parts of the body through a vast network of veins. The valve between the right atrium and the right ventricle opens and blood flows into the ventricle. The ventricle has thick, muscular walls that contract and force the blood out of the heart through a large artery called the *pulmonary artery.* Through this artery, the blood goes to the lungs, where the blood cells take on oxygen. The blood then moves back to the heart through the *pulmonary veins,* entering the left atrium. Again the blood

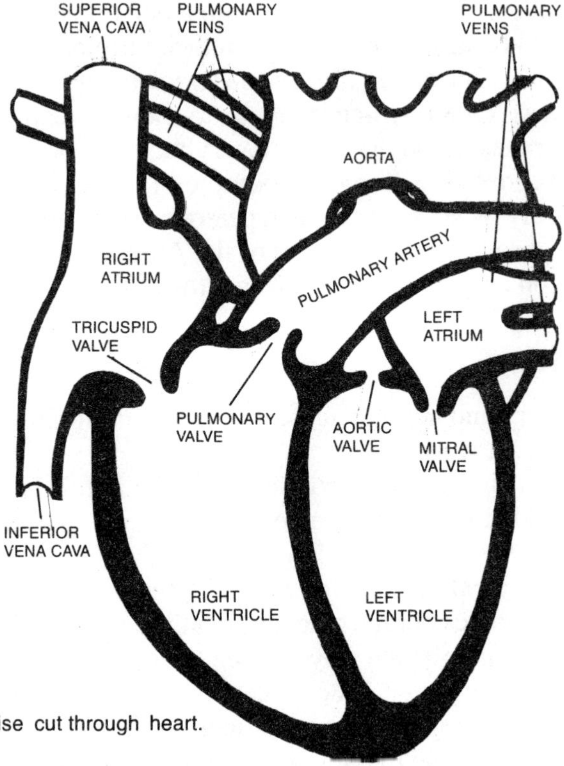

Lengthwise cut through heart.

passes through a valve, flowing down into the left ventricle. As the left ventricle contracts, it pumps blood into a large artery called the *aorta.* This artery takes the blood, via a network of increasingly smaller arteries, to all parts of the body.

With each heartbeat, the left ventricle sends into the arteries approximately 2½ ounces of blood. In an adult, the heart beats 60 to 90 times a minute—more than 85,000 beats a day. In children, the heart beats faster—100 to 120 times a minute, or more than 140,000 times a day. Your heart beats before you are born and never stops until you die. The heart muscle rests a fraction of a second between beats. That is all the rest the heart gets or needs.

The Coronary Arteries

A muscle needs nourishment and oxygen, and the heart is no exception. Nourishment and oxygen are brought to all parts of the body in the blood that flows through the arteries. The heart has its own set of arteries to supply it with blood. These arteries, called *coronary arteries,* bring to the heart muscle fuel to furnish energy and oxygen to burn the fuel, and muscle material for repair. They carry away the waste, and they are essential for the life and activity of the heart. These coronary arteries branch out from the base of the aorta just as it leaves the left chamber of the heart and just above the valve that separates the aorta from the ventricle. They and the network of vessels branching off of them come down over the top of the heart like a crown (corona). They are the most important blood vessels in the body. Leakage, blockage, or bursting of weakened coronary blood vessels almost surely leads to death.

Coronary arteries that become blocked are diseased. A healthy artery, with blood flowing rapidly through it, will not become blocked. The disease that affects coronary arteries is *atherosclerosis,* also called hardening of the arteries, a condition in which the walls of the arteries become less elastic ("hard") because they are coated with a fatty deposit. The fatty deposit not only hardens the artery's wall but also narrows its inside diameter. The narrowed artery can carry less blood than a healthy one. Also, the fatty deposit roughens the artery walls, which slows the flow of blood. Clots may form in blood that flows slowly. Such a clot, trying to move through a narrowed artery, may block it, cutting off all flow of blood through it. The tissue that was supplied with blood flowing through the artery then dies. This can happen in any artery, but if it happens in a coronary artery, a heart attack follows. Doctors call this type of heart attack a *coronary thrombosis*. It is the most common type of heart attack and can happen at any time—during sleep as well as during normal daily activity.

A heart attack can also occur if the flow of blood is stopped, not by a clot, but by fatty deposits completely filling the artery.

Either way, the attack may be so mild that the victim does not even notice it (although this is very rare), or it may be very severe and even bring death. How serious a heart attack is depends on how much of the heart muscle is damaged by sudden blood starvation. The damaged or dead region of the heart is called a *myocardial infarct*.

The body has its own remarkable way of averting disaster even though coronary arteries are hardening. Branches of arteries neighboring the one that is hardening carry more blood than they formerly did, thus taking over the work of the diseased artery. Also, new arterial branches may form and carry blood to those parts of the heart that need it. This explains why persons with hardening of the arteries do not always suffer heart attacks or even experience pain when the diseased artery becomes blocked. The taking over of blood circulation by auxiliary or newly formed arteries is called

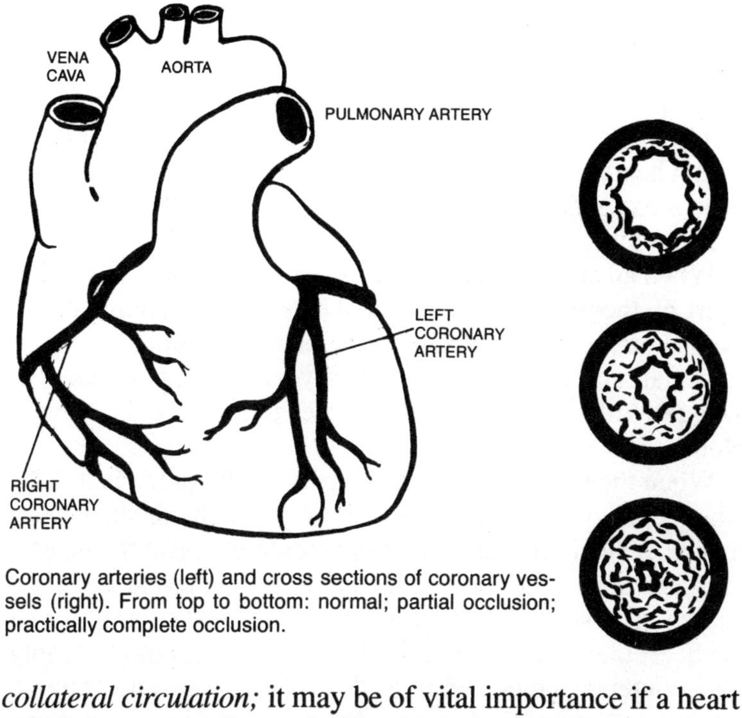

Coronary arteries (left) and cross sections of coronary vessels (right). From top to bottom: normal; partial occlusion; practically complete occlusion.

collateral circulation; it may be of vital importance if a heart attack does occur. It may help to keep the victim alive during the first few hours after the attack. Then it can help the heart to repair itself and regain its normal strength.

Angina Pectoris and Congestive Heart Failure

If there is a discrepancy between the supply and demand of oxygen to the heart, severe chest pain may result. The discrepancy can be caused by low oxygen levels in the blood because of smoking or respiratory disease, or it may be caused by diseased coronary arteries. These chest pains are called *angina pectoris* and in most cases are a chronic condition. An attack of angina pectoris is not to be confused with a heart attack. However, if there is a prolonged severe lack of oxygenated blood to a part of the heart, it can lead to a heart attack.

When an angina pectoris attack occurs, the demand on the heart by the rest of the body must be reduced. Complete, even short, rest from whatever the patient is doing is essential, and medication (a nitroglycerine pill put under the tongue) will help to dilate the arteries to improve the flow of blood.

When the heart has to pump harder all the time, as it does when a person has atherosclerosis, or when he or she is very much overweight, the heart muscle enlarges. But the heart muscle can enlarge just so much before the muscle fibers stretch. The stretched muscle is weaker. Each contraction of the heart then pumps less blood. The ventricles fail to empty their contents of blood entirely. This causes a backup of blood into the vessels of the lungs and poor circulation throughout the body. As the heart pump becomes more and more ineffectual, it fails to return blood from the feet and legs, and the blood begins to collect there. As a result, the ankles become swollen. When the heart becomes weaker, blood may collect in the thighs, abdomen, and lungs. The victim becomes very easily fatigued and suffers shortness of breath, at first during exertion, and then even when at rest. The shortness of breath, followed by gasping, may come on as an attack. This is called *congestive heart failure*. It can be a direct result of high blood pressure.

Who Will Have a Heart Attack?

Physicians cannot say exactly who will have a heart attack, but they do know that certain *risk factors* increase the likelihood of occurrence.

Risk Factor 1: High Blood Pressure (Hypertension)

High blood pressure, or hypertension, is a major risk factor in heart attacks. It speeds up hardening of the arteries, especially the coronary arteries. We have seen how narrowing of these arteries can lead directly to heart attack.

High blood pressure afflicts about 15 percent of people in the United States. It is called a "silent killer" because it is not recognizable by its victim in the early stages. Once high blood pressure is recognized, it usually can be brought under control by use of medicine and a diet prescribed by a physician. Heart specialists too often find that victims of a heart attack had been told previously by a physician that they had high blood pressure but had not followed doctor's orders to diet or take medication. They had not taken the disease seriously.

As a direct cause of heart attacks, high blood pressure should never be ignored.

Risk Factor 2: High Blood-fat Levels

Fats carried in the blood are called *lipids*. They build fatty tissue in the body and are sources of energy. Lipids seem to be able to adhere to the inside walls of arteries and build up fatty deposits that narrow the blood vessel. It is not clear just how this takes place, but experiments with animals have proved that increase in lipids in the blood leads to hardening of the arteries.

Two kinds of lipids are involved in this disease: *cholesterol* and *triglycerides*. High levels of cholesterol are found in egg yolks, saturated fats, the inner organs of animals such as brain and liver, and shellfish. The body converts carbohydrates such as sugar, flour, cornmeal, and rice into triglycerides. Eating foods low in cholesterol and avoiding as much as possible foods that will convert into triglycerides will lower the risk factor of high blood-fat levels.

Risk Factor 3: Low Level of HDL and High Level of LDL

Lipids do not float freely in the bloodstream; they are bound to proteins. There are high-density lipoproteins (HDL) and low-density lipoproteins (LDL). Every person has these in his or her blood. HDL is composed of almost 50 percent protein and less than 25 percent cholesterol, whereas LDL is almost 50 percent cholesterol and 25 percent protein. Obviously, it is better to have a high level of HDL and a low level of LDL than the reverse, which would increase the amount of blood fats.

Stopping smoking, taking up regular moderate exercise, and eating a diet rich in fish, vegetable oils, and skim milk can lower LDL levels, thus contributing to a decrease in the risk of heart disease.

Risk Factor 4: Diabetes

In Framingham, Massachusetts, for thirty years there has been a continuing study of several aspects of the health of citizens. The study has shown that one of every two diabetics suffers from coronary heart disease. This finding should warn every untreated diabetic of the grave risk he or she is running. Not only the coronary arteries, but other blood vessels in diabetics may be diseased. The risk is twice as great for diabetics as for the rest of the population, and the risk is greater for women than men.

Risk Factor 5: High Uric Acid Levels in the Blood

Coronary heart disease is three times as frequent in persons with both high blood pressure and high levels of uric acid in the blood as it is in those with high blood pressure alone. However, it is not known just why blood uric acid should be associated with coronary heart disease.

Risk Factor 6: Overweight

Studies have not shown that overweight itself is a risk factor in heart attacks. However, 85 percent of persons with diabetes, 60 percent of persons with high blood pressure, and 80 percent of persons with abnormal fat metabolism are overweight. Thus, overweight could be a contributing risk in heart attacks.

However, angina pectoris is five times as common among overweight persons as among those of ideal weight. Thus, overweight is a definite risk factor for angina.

Risk Factor 7: Cigarette Smoking

Coronary heart disease is three times as common among cigarette smokers as among nonsmokers, ex-smokers, or cigar and pipe smokers who do not inhale. Therefore smoking is a high risk factor for heart attacks.

It is encouraging to hear that the risk for heart attack for ex-smokers a few years after the habit has been kicked is nearly as low as that for people who have never smoked. The average age for the first heart attack among nonsmokers is 63, but it is 53 among cigarette smokers. Smoking cigarettes is also the most important factor in bringing on a second heart attack and death.

Risk Factor 8: Lack of Exercise

There is no direct proof that lack of exercise is an important risk factor in heart attacks. "Lack of exercise" means the life-style of persons who work sitting down and whose recreation also involves sitting (at a bar or in front of a television set). However, there is clear evidence that persons active in sports have less coronary disease and heart attacks. Also, these active persons are less likely to develop fatal complications within 48 hours after a heart attack.

Risk Factor 9: Heredity

Although heart attacks are not hereditary, it seems that heredity is an indirect risk factor; there is a likelihood that it plays an important role in atherosclerosis, high blood pressure, high blood-fat levels, and diabetes, all possible causes of heart attack. As far as high fat levels in the blood are concerned, there is a well-known hereditary disease (hypercholesterolemia) that causes high LDL and has been known to wipe out whole families. This is another reason to consider heredity as being associated with heart disease.

Risk Factor 10: Contraceptive Pills

Taking the contraceptive pill does not seem to be a risk factor in itself; however, in combination with one or more of the risk factors described before, it may become an additional risk factor. In such cases, a woman who has taken the pill for a number of years should have regular heart checkups.

Risk Factor 11: Stress and Personality

A high percentage of patients questioned about what they believed to be the cause of their heart attacks answered, "Stress." Stress is not a clear-cut concept, so it is very difficult to decide whether it really is a risk factor in heart attacks. There are, however, people who seem to live under "stress" all the time. This type of personality is impatient of others and himself, lives by the clock, strives to outdo others, cannot have fun without feeling guilty, and cannot listen to others without constantly interrupting. Some studies, which have not gone unchallenged, show that this type of person is "coronary-prone," having more than twice as great a chance of having a heart attack as most other personality types.

Can Heart Attacks Be Prevented?

The answer probably is no. But the chances of having a heart attack certainly can be lowered by eliminating as many risk factors from one's life as possible. It is never too late to

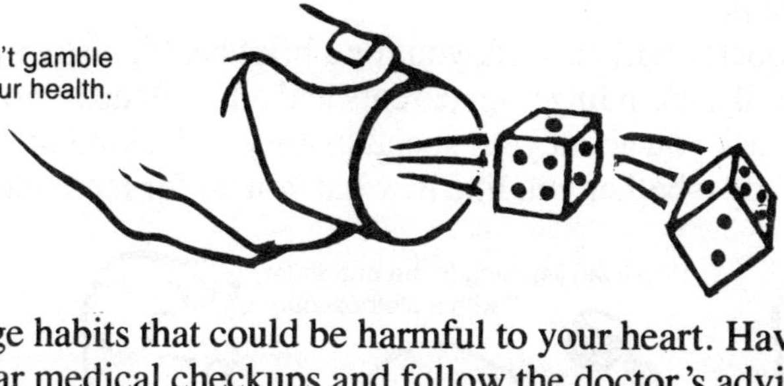

Don't gamble with your health.

change habits that could be harmful to your heart. Have regular medical checkups and follow the doctor's advice about coronary risk factors, including treatment of high blood pressure, avoiding foods high in cholesterol and saturated fats, and stopping smoking.

Diagnosis of a Heart Condition

Every thorough physical examination includes tests that provide the physician with information on how the patient's heart is functioning. Everyone should have physical examinations at regular intervals—at least once a year even if feeling well.

The examination by a physician is especially important if mild symptoms of angina pectoris have occurred and disappeared. Do *not* think that you do not need medical help because the symptoms went away by themselves.

The examination for diagnosing heart symptoms begins like the examination for any complaint that is taken to a physician. You will be asked a number of questions about your present health and your past illnesses. The doctor will want to know what brought you to the office, whether you have any specific complaints, or, if this is a routine visit, what is the usual state of your health and what, if anything, is different now.

The doctor will also ask you for a brief health history of your family, including your parents and other blood relatives. He may ask you about your social history—the kind of work you do and whether you like it, what you do for recreation,

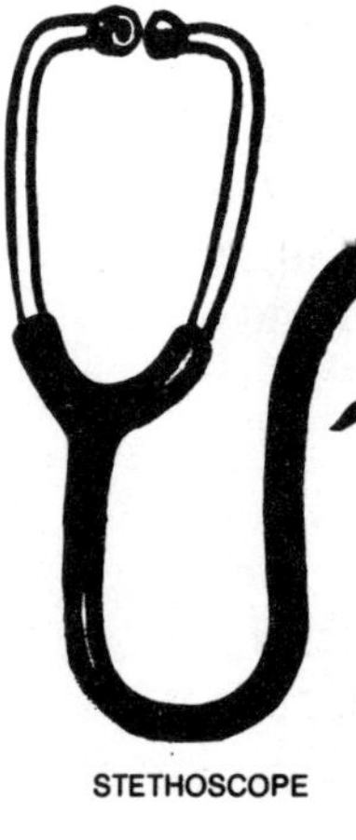

Physician listening to the heartbeat with a stethoscope.

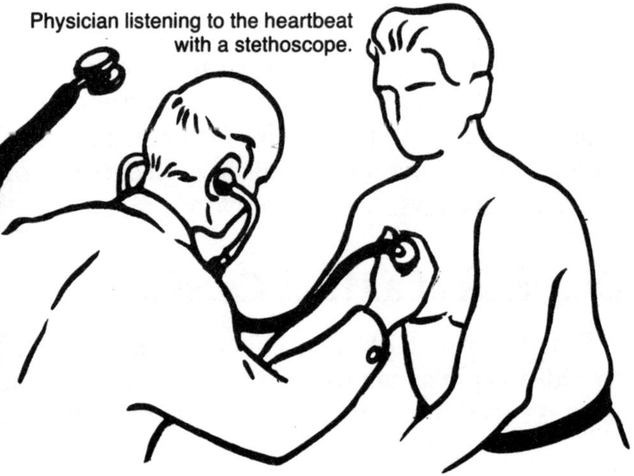

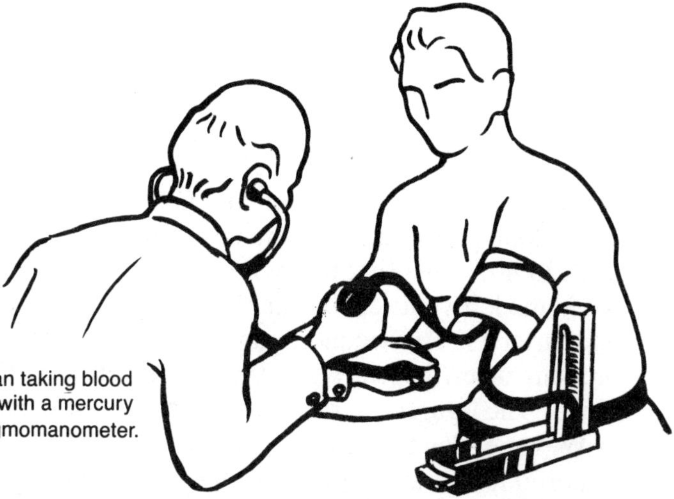

Physician taking blood pressure with a mercury column sphygmomanometer.

what education you have had, and what kind of family life you have. These questions are designed to give him a picture of your life-style, especially habits that might be risk factors for heart or blood-vessel disease.

The doctor will measure your height and weight. Your weight in relation to your height will tell him whether you are overweight.

The doctor will take your body temperature, check your breathing, and take your pulse. The pulse will tell him how many times a minute your heart is beating. He will be able to tell from the rate of your pulse whether your heart is beating regularly. The pulse is usually taken at one wrist, but to find out how well the heart is pumping blood to all parts of the body, the doctor may also feel the pulse at your throat, near your right and left collarbones, and at your ankles.

To double check the regularity or irregularities of the heartbeat that might have been revealed by feeling the pulse, and to check whether the heart valves are working properly, he will listen to the heartbeat with a stethoscope. This instrument magnifies the sounds of the heart.

The physician will measure your blood pressure with an instrument called a sphygmomanometer. It shows the level of your blood pressure in millimeters of mercury, for example, as "120/80." This first figure represents your blood pressure when the left ventricle of your heart is pumping blood into your arteries. The second figure represents your blood pressure when the heart is resting and the atria are filling with blood. The figures are read "one-twenty over eighty."

We have seen that the level of blood fat represents an important risk factor. So the doctor will probably order blood tests that will show the levels of cholesterol and triglycerides in your blood. Another blood test will show the amount of glucose, or blood sugar. A high amount of blood sugar may indicate that you have diabetes mellitus, another high risk factor for heart attack.

An X ray of your chest shows whether your heart has become enlarged. A larger-than-normal heart may indicate that the heart has been overworking in order to pump blood through arteries that are being clogged by fatty deposits. In addition to taking an X ray, the doctor may use a fluoroscope, a kind of X ray in which the parts inside your body show up on a screen somewhat like a large television screen. Fluoroscopy enables the doctor to see the heart in motion as it beats.

Besides listening to the heart through a stethoscope and seeing it by means of X rays, there are complicated instruments that can give a physician valuable information directly from the heart. One of these is the electrocardiograph. This instrument measures the electric currents generated by the heart and records them as a jagged line on a long strip of paper called an electrocardiogram (ECG or EKG). The ECG reveals to the doctor irregular heart rhythms, which can indicate heart disease or damage to the heart from small or large attacks of angina pectoris.

To make an electrocardiogram, the doctor places small rubber suction cups at several places on the patient's chest. In these cups are wires that conduct the electrical impulses produced by the beating heart to the electrocardiograph. The instrument converts the electrical impulses into lines on the strip of paper. When the procedure is done with the patient lying down, the electrocardiogram is called a resting ECG. The recording can also be made during exercise; it is then called an exercise ECG or a "stress test." It shows the electrical impulses of the heart while the patient is jogging on a treadmill, walking up and down a short flight of stairs, or pedaling a stationary bicycle.

If the doctor wants an ECG that is recorded over a longer period of time than just a few minutes in an office or clinic, a portable electrocardiograph may be used. This instrument is no larger than some portable radios. A wire runs from the instrument through the patient's clothing to the chest. The electrocardiograph is carried by the patient for 24 hours, thus providing a record of heart activity while the patient is working, eating, sleeping, and engaging in other everyday activities, including situations of stress should they occur.

Instead of a stethoscope, the physician can use a phonocardiograph, which transmits the sounds of the heart through microphones placed on the chest of the patient into sensitive recording equipment. In this way the doctor can listen to the sounds again and compare them to the sounds of the heart recorded at a later time.

After the doctor has diagnosed a diseased heart, cardiac catheterization may be necessary. A catheter is a thin flexible tube that can be introduced into a body organ. A cardiac catheter is made of materials to which blood does not adhere, such as woven plastic. It is inserted into a vein or artery (usually of a leg or arm) and gently threaded through the blood vessel to the heart while the doctor watches its progress with a fluoroscope.

Blood samples from inside the heart can be withdrawn through the catheter for laboratory analysis. Blood pressure in the individual heart chambers, across heart valves, or in the aorta and vena cava can be measured. So can the rate at which the heart is pumping blood.

Cardiac catheterization requires that the patient be hospitalized for two or three days, as it can be done only under local anesthesia and the patient must be kept under observation for a short period afterwards.

More knowledge of the heart activity and condition of the blood vessels can be acquired by angiocardiography. Angiocardiography is done by injecting into the bloodstream certain radioisotopes, substances that are slightly radioactive for a few hours. Using a sensitive device called a gamma-scanner, the physician can detect and record the tiny amounts of radioactivity emitted as the radioisotopes circulate through the heart chamber and large blood vessels. The records, called scans, aid the doctor in evaluating such factors as blood supply to the heart, size of the heart, amount of blood pumped per beat, and extent of any damage to the heart muscle.

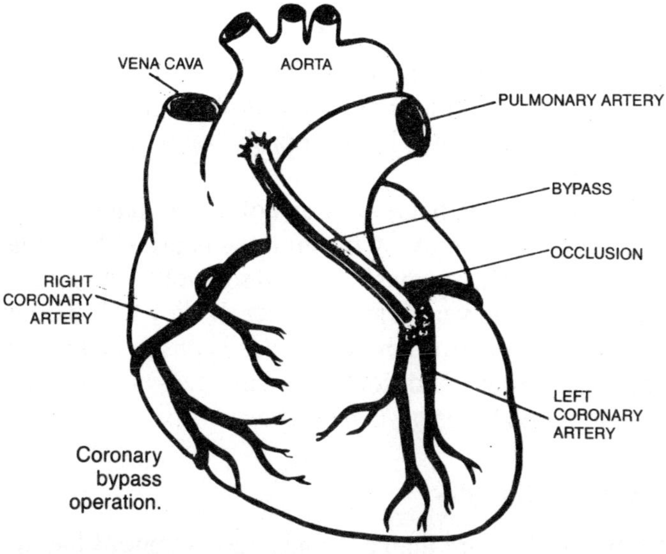

Coronary bypass operation.

Surgical Help

In some instances surgery is necessary to restore a damaged heart or blood vessel.

When the coronary arteries are so narrowed that the flow of the oxygen-containing blood to the heart is dangerously impaired, a *coronary bypass* operation may be required. This involves constructing detours through which blood can flow, bypassing the narrowed sections of coronary arteries to keep the heart muscle supplied. Veins or arteries taken from other parts of the body where they are not essential are grafted onto the heart to construct these bypasses.

In some cases a patient develops an *aneurysm*. This is a ballooning out of the wall of a vein, an artery, or the heart because of weakening of the wall by disease or an abnormality present at birth. If the aneurysm is tiny, it will be left alone, and it may diminish in size as the heart or blood vessels become healthier due to a good program of health care. If the aneurysm is large, it probably will have to be removed by surgery.

The valves in the heart are flaps of tissue that prevent backflow of blood moving through the heart and circulatory system. These valves must close completely for a split second before the ventricles contract. If they fail to do this, some of the blood from the ventricles is pushed back into the atria, a dangerous condition. The damaged valve or valves can be repaired by *open-heart surgery.*

Open-heart Surgery

Until a little more than a decade ago, surgeons had to operate on the heart while it continued its pumping action. This limited them to operations that did not involve opening the ventricles. The developmentof the *heart-lung machine* has made it possible for surgeons to open the heart and make needed repairs. It can take over the work of heart and lungs for a certain period of time while open-heart surgery is performed.

In use of this machine, the two large veins that return blood from the upper and lower body to the right atrium are tied off and connected in a way that causes the blood from all the veins to flow directly into the heart-lung machine. The machine contains a pump that takes over the pumping action of the heart. As blood passes through the machine, oxygen is added to it as the lungs would normally do. This oxygenated blood is pumped back into the body through connections to one or more of the major branches of the aorta. One branch must go to the heart, because the heart tissue must continue to be supplied with oxygen or it will die.

Once all the connections have been made, the heart-lung machine takes over the functions of heart and lungs. It is not even necessary for the body to continue respiration. The surgeon now has a few hours in which to open the heart and work on it.

The heart-lung machine is a great advance in heart surgery; however, it has a few drawbacks. One is that after surgery many patients have a temporary period of mental imbalance.

Heart Transplants

A physician specializing in heart disease may find that a heart, following a heart attack, is in such bad condition that neither surgery nor any other form of treatment will make it function normally. As a last resort, a heart transplant may be performed.

Transplanting parts of the body from one person to another is not a new technique. If one considers blood as an organ, it has been transplanted from one person to another in blood transfusions. Early in the history of blood transfusion, it was recognized that the blood of one person could not always be transfused into the bloodstream of another. Looking for the reason, medical scientists found that there are different types of blood. They also found that one type mixed with another could cause an allergy-like reaction in which the red blood cells clumped together.

The first organ transplants were the replacement of diseased arteries. For example, a healthy section of the aorta of a person who had died in an accident could be used to replace the diseased section of the aorta of another person. Sometimes the replacement was not successful because the replacement blood vessel would not grow as part of the body into which it had been placed. This happened because the body rejected the new organ. The body's system that enables it to develop immunity to infectious diseases rejected the new organ as if it were an invading bacterium. Ways were found in some cases to temporarily suppress the working of the immune system, and the transplants were successful. Kidneys, livers, and other organs have been transplanted.

It was only a next step until the transplantation of a heart was attempted. The first successful heart transplant was performed in 1968. Since then more than 200 have been performed. The patient's heart is removed, but the back of the right and left atria are left in the chest cavity. Then the back of the right and left atria of the donor's heart are removed. Finally, the donor's heart is fitted to what is left of the patient's heart, and the two are sewn together.

The survival rate of heart transplant patients today is seven out of ten. However, heart transplantation will have only limited use because there will always be a short supply of donors' hearts and few people will be willing to risk the surgery.

Pacemaker

The rhythm of the heartbeat is controlled by a small mass of specialized cells embedded in the roof of the right atrium. These cells give rise to electrical impulses that initiate contractions of the heart. The cells are called the sinoatrial node of Keith-Flack, or the *pacemaker*. Sometimes, if the pacemaker is damaged, other heart tissues in the ventricles

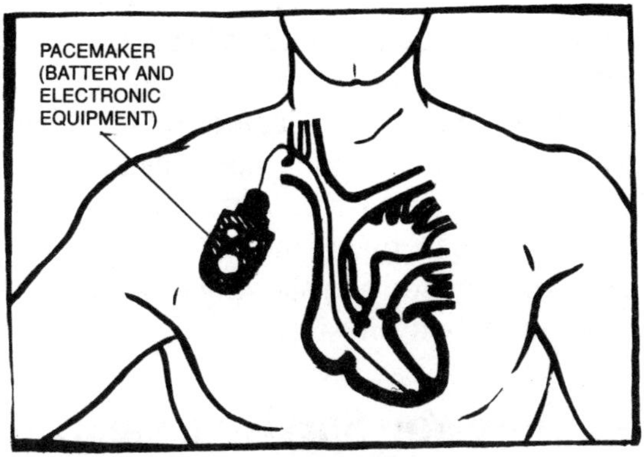

An implanted
artificial pacemaker.

themselves can take over the role of the pacemaker. The ventricles receive their signals from the pacemaker via two nerves, one for each ventricle.

If any damage occurs to the pacemaker or the nerves connecting it to the ventricles, the heart may stop beating. This is called a *heart blockage*. A patient whose pacemaker is damaged may not experience a total blockage, but a reduction in the number of heartbeats per minute. He must be taken immediately to a hospital, where a wire is placed in his heart through a vein opened at the neck. The wire is attached to a device that sends electric impulses to the heart at proper intervals. This device is an artificial pacemaker.

After a few days, a portable pacemaker will replace the stationary one. It may be worn by the patient wherever he or she goes. It is powered by a small electric cell, or battery, in a plastic case that is implanted under the skin. The tiny battery that powers the pacemaker continues to produce electric current for years, but eventually it runs down. Then a physician will perform a minor surgical operation in which he replaces the whole pacemaker. The French have devised an atomic-powered pacemaker that can last ten years, but it is extremely expensive.

Patients who wear pacemakers must have them monitored by a physician at regular intervals to check that the batteries are not becoming weak. Between checkups patients can check their pacemaker themselves by taking their pulse twice a day. If they notice a slowing down of the heartbeat, they must go to their physician.

Suppose You Survive a Heart Attack

You have had a heart attack and have gotten to the hospital alive. You will be rushed to the intensive care unit, which has many kinds of equipment that will be used to keep you alive during the very critical time right after a heart attack. There is oxygen that can be pumped into your lungs so that your body tissues, especially your brain, stay alive. There are drugs that can help to get your damaged heart back to regular beating. Your "vital signs" (temperature, respiration, heart rate, and blood pressure) are constantly observed and recorded. When these emergency procedures are no longer required, you will be transferred from the intensive care unit to a regular hospital rooom.

The Road Back

With prompt and proper care the heart begins to heal. As the heart heals, scar tissue forms at the damaged area. The recovery time for heart attack patients varies, depending on the extent of the injury to the heart muscle and the occurrence of complications.

It was formerly believed that heart patients needed long periods of bed rest. At present, physicians agree that it is beneficial for the patient to get out of bed as soon as possible. A rehabilitation program is begun while the patient is still hospitalized. A nurse or physical therapist begins to work with the patient twice a day, if possible. The patient is taught breathing and relaxation exercises and then given active and passive exercises for the arm and leg muscles.

After exercising still more muscles while lying in bed or sitting up, the patient is allowed to walk around the room, go to the bathroom, and eat at a table. Little by little the patient is allowed to do more strenuous exercises, walk a little farther, and slowly climb stairs. Eventually the patient is able to participate in gymnastic groups that perform exercises especially designed for persons who have had coronary attacks.

Emotional Reaction to Heart Attacks

The seriousness of a heart attack is misunderstood by very few patients. Although most understand that they have come very close to death and probably must face the possibility of death until they have fully recovered, they are usually unwilling to talk about their fears. A result of suppressing these fears is that the patient becomes depressed. An experienced heart specialist may be able to see the onset of the depression and prescribe antidepressant drugs. It is much better, however, if a patient can bring himself or herself to talk of these fears with family members.

A narrow escape from death produces fear in everyone. In the days and weeks of inactivity that pass following a heart attack, every patient goes through a period in which the fear of death is replaced by a fear of life. The patient asks, "How shall life continue?"

Patients who face this question squarely and make no attempt to evade the difficulties that must follow a serious heart attack are likely to make a new and happy life for themselves. Those who evade the question make a miserable future for themselves and may even bring on a new heart attack.

Life-style Gains

By the time a heart attack patient leaves the hospital, he or she has had a chance to make some gains that partly offset the fear and anxiety produced by the attack. If he or she has been a smoker, smoking has been forbidden for weeks, and with that time as a head start the patient should be able to kick the smoking habit altogether. Also, the overweight patient will have lost weight. This problem thus has also been licked if the convalescent is able to maintain his new trimness. Anybody who regularly drank alcohol will not have done so during his or her stay in the hospital. Again, the patient has a head start. Among the reasons for not drinking are that alcohol is high in calories and should be shunned by the patient who is trying to keep a trim weight. Furthermore, it has been found that, although alcohol increases the amount of blood pumped by the hearts of healthy persons, for some unknown reason it diminishes the amount of blood pumped in persons who have had heart attacks.

A heart patient not suffering from angina pectoris and not prone to heart failure can, by a planned program of gradually increased physical exercise and activity, make the heart as strong as it was before the attack or even stronger. This has the psychological side-effect that he or she begins to feel much more self-assured.

Some patients feel that the heart attack has propelled them into early old age, and they cannot face this prospect. They reject the doctor's advice to take life easier than before the attack, and they drop the schedule of medication that has been worked out for them. In short, they try to pretend that they are not recovering from a nearly fatal illness. The usual result is a second coronary attack, which, if not fatal, will show them how wrong their attitude was.

Another type of coronary convalescent keeps in mind his or her recent brush with death and fears that it is still just around the corner. This type of person pities and overprotects himself or herself and becomes very selfish, demanding that others be constantly aware of his problems. He or she fears returning to employment and decides not to do so, thus becoming a burden on the immediate family and possibly on society.

Most patients can and should return to work. Some may have to change occupation or alter their life-style. Continued guidance and management by the doctor is important. It varies for each individual and usually follows a long-term health plan that the doctor draws up for his patient.

Other patients also may decide not to return to work because they had wanted to drop out of society for a long time, and the heart attack gave them an excuse to do so. They, too, may need professional psychological counseling or therapy to be guided back to assuming a responsible place in society.

Another type of cardiac convalescent keeps in mind the health gains he or she obtained when in crisis and early convalescence and determines to retain them. Also, this patient takes the time given by convalescence to review his or her former life-style and decide whether it was worthwhile. If it involved great ambition and consequent stress, the convalescent, realizing that he or she cannot go back to these things without risk of another heart attack, will choose a way of life that is slower but may be richer in personal rewards because it allows time to enjoy many things that there never seemed to be time for previously. Such heart attack convalescents can lead normal lives of normal length.

Heart Disease and Sex

An important aspect in the life of patients with heart disease may unfortunately be passed over by many physicians. This aspect is the patient's sex life. Since sexual activity creates a heavy work load on any person's heart, it is an especially important factor for a heart patient.

Many patients have their first heart attack during sexual activity. Sometimes the first severe chest pains that are signs of coronary atherosclerosis occur during sexual intercourse. Thus, anyone experiencing any kind of chest pains during sexual activity should report them to a physician. Also, many recuperating patients are obliged to return to the hospital because they have engaged in sex too soon after their release. It makes little sense to follow a doctor's orders to engage in only very light exertion, such as a leisurely walk, and then return home to the extraordinary exertion of sexual intercourse. This does not mean that a person who has had a heart attack must refrain from sex. It does mean that he or she must first strengthen his or her body, including the heart. When a patient has achieved vigorous general health, he or she may resume sexual activity. A patient who follows his physician's prescriptions for strengthening the heart and body after a heart attack usually can resume sexual activity about three months after leaving the hospital.

Since pregnancy involves an increased work load for the heart, women with a history of such diseases as high blood pressure, rheumatic fever, thyroid disease, atherosclerosis, and others are usually discouraged by their physicians from becoming pregnant. In such cases, more than the opinion of an obstetrician should be sought. A heart specialist should be consulted also.

Heart Drugs

Most patients recovering from a heart attack will have to take some kind of medicine for quite a while, if not for the rest of their lives. It is important to have some knowledge of such drugs, especially of the specific drugs that were prescribed. The situation might occur when the patient has to travel and his doctor is not available by telephone when difficulties arise. It is also possible that the patient may lose the prescribed drugs and need to tell a strange doctor what drugs were prescribed for him.

Digitalis, a drug prepared from leaves of the foxglove plant, and its derivatives are commonly used heart drugs. Digitalis causes a more forceful contraction of the heart muscle and regulates the speed of transmission of electrical impulses in the heart. Patients taking digitalis drugs should follow the dosage prescribed by their physicians very carefully. Overdosing with digitalis may result in heart failure, the very ailment the drug is prescribed to prevent.

Pronestyl and quinidine are prescribed for irregular or rapid heartbeats and for premature beats. A dose of these drugs lasts four to six hours, but the commercial preparations, Quinidex, Quinaglute, and Cardioquin, have longer-lasting effects.

Anticoagulants are used to prevent or delay the formation of blood clots in any of the blood vessels. Some anticoagulants in pill form are Dicumarol, Coumadin, Panwarfin, Sintrom, and Liquamar, all of which are commercial preparations. If an anticoagulant is given by injection, it probably will be heparin. Anticoagulants may have undesirable side-effects, so their use should be carefully watched by a physician.

Diuretics are drugs that aid the kidneys in increasing the amount of sodium excreted in the urine. They are used to treat heart failure and hypertension. Diuretics are sometimes called "water pills" or "dehydrating pills."

Although it may be desirable to eliminate sodium from the body, diuretics also eliminate potassium, which is needed by the cells of the body. To counteract the loss, the patient if so ordered can use potassium chloride salt as a substitute for sodium chloride, which is table salt. Also, bananas, citrus fruits and juices, and tomato juice all have a high potassium content and may be eaten to replace the lost potassium.

Nitroglycerine is very effective in stopping the pain of angina pectoris. It is usually given in the form of a small white pill that is placed under the tongue and allowed to dissolve when an attack of angina begins.

Nitroglycerine is a very unstable drug. Even moderate heat will destroy it. One should not leave a bottle of nitroglycerine tablets on the bathroom windowsill where the sun can reach it; nor should it be left in the glove compartment of a car in summer. A patient can tell if the pills are losing their strength because more will be required to produce the same relief.